Evidence-based Medicine Toolkit

Carl Heneghan
and
Douglas Badenoch

Centre for Evidence-based Medicine,
Nuffield Department of Clinical Medicine,
John Radcliffe Hospital, Headington, Oxford

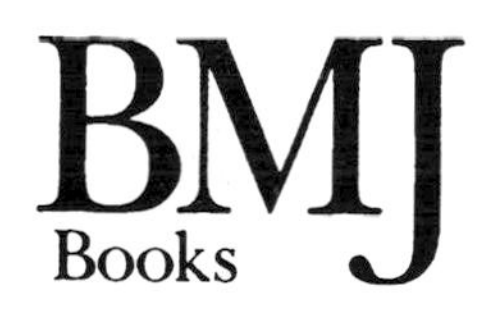

BMJ Books is an imprint of the BMJ Publishing Group

First published in 2002
by BMJ Books, BMA House, Tavistock Square,
London WC1H 9JR

www.bmjbooks.com

British Library Cataloguing in Publication Data

A catalogue record for this book is available
from the British Library

ISBN 0 7279 1601 7

Typeset by Newgen Imaging Systems Pvt. Ltd.
Printed and bound in Spain by GraphyCems, Navarra

Contents

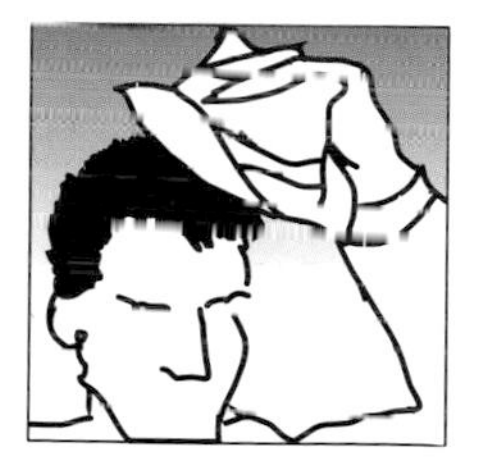

This handbook was compiled by Carl Heneghan and Douglas Badenoch. The materials have largely been adapted from previous work by those who know better than us, especially other members of the Centre for Evidence-based Medicine (Chris Ball, Martin Dawes, Jonathan Mant, Bob Phillips, David Sackett, Kate Seers, Sharon Straus) and CASPfew (Steve Ashwell, Anne Brice, Andre Tomlin).

Introduction

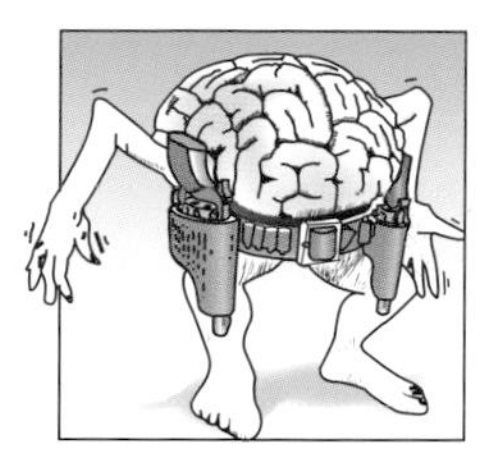

This "toolkit" is designed as a summary and reminder of the key elements of practising evidence-based medicine (EBM). It has largely been adapted from resources developed at the Centre for Evidence-based Medicine. For more detailed coverage, you should refer to the other EBM texts and web pages cited throughout.

The first page of each chapter presents a "minimalist" checklist of the key points. Further sections within each chapter address these points in more detail and give additional background information. Ideally, you should just need to refer to the first page to get the basics, and delve into the further sections as required.

Occasionally, you will see the dustbin icon on the right. This means that the question being discussed is a "filter" question for critical appraisal: if the answer is not satisfactory, you should consider ditching the paper and looking elsewhere. If you don't ditch the paper, you should be aware that the effect it describes may not appear in your patient in the same way.

Definition of Evidence-based Medicine

Evidence based Medicine is the "conscientious, explicit and judicious use of current best evidence in making decisions about individual patients". This means "integrating individual clinical expertise with the best available external clinical evidence from systematic research".[1]

We can summarise the EBM approach as a five-step model:

1. Asking answerable clinical questions.
2. Searching for the evidence.
3. Critically appraising the evidence for its validity and relevance.
4. Making a decision, by integrating the evidence with your clinical expertise and the patient's values.
5. Evaluating your performance.

Reference

1. Sackett DL *et al.* Evidence based medicine: what it is and what it isn't. *BMJ* 1996;**312**:71–2.

Asking answerable questions

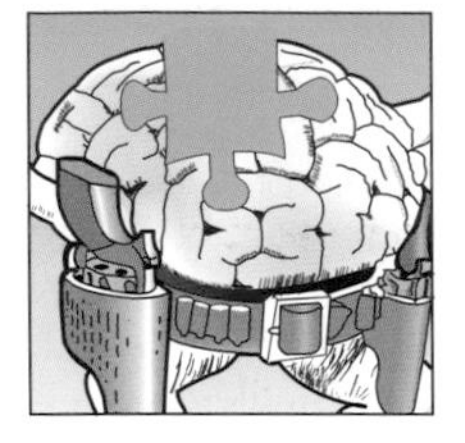

The four main elements of a well-formed clinical question are:

1. **P**atient or Problem
2. **I**ntervention
3. **C**omparison intervention (if appropriate)
4. **O**utcome(s)

Element	Tips	Specific example
Patient or Problem	Starting with your patient ask "How would I describe a group of patients similar to mine?"	"In women over 40 with heart failure from dilated cardiomyopathy ..."
Intervention	Ask "Which main intervention am I considering?"	"... would adding anticoagulation with warfarin to standard heart failure therapy..."
Comparison intervention	Ask "What is the main alternative to compare with the intervention?"	"... when compared with standard therapy alone ..."
Outcome	Ask "What can I hope to accomplish?" or "What could this exposure really affect?"	"... lead to lower mortality or morbidity from thromboembolism."

The terms you identify from this process will form the basis of your search for evidence and the question as your guide in assessing its relevance.

Bear in mind that how specific you are will affect the outcome of your search: general terms (such as "heart failure") will give you a broad search, while more specific terms (for example, "congestive heart failure") will narrow the search. Also, you should think about alternative ways or aspects of describing your question (for example, New York Heart Association Classification).

Patient or problem

Firstly, think about the patient and/or setting you are dealing with. Try to identify all of the clinical characteristics which influence the problem, which are relevant to your practice and which would affect the relevance of research you might find. It will help your search if you can be as specific as possible at this stage, but you should bear in mind that if you are too narrow in searching you may miss important articles (see next section).

Intervention

Next, think about what you are considering doing. In therapy, this may be a drug or counselling; in diagnosis it could be a test or screening programme. If your question is about harm or aetiology, it may be exposure to an environmental agent. Again, it pays to be specific when describing the intervention, as you will want to reflect what is possible in your practice. If considering drug treatment, for example, dosage and delivery should be included. Again, you can always broaden your search later if your question is too narrow.

Comparison intervention

What would you do if you didn't perform the intervention? This might be nothing, or standard care, but you should think at this stage about the alternatives. There may be useful evidence which directly compares the two interventions. Even if there isn't, this will remind you that any evidence on the intervention should be interpreted in the context of what your normal practice would be.

Outcome

There is an important distinction to be made between the outcome that is relevant to your patient or problem and the outcome measures deployed in studies. You should spend some time working out exactly what outcome is important to you, your patient, and the time-frame which is appropriate. In serious diseases it is often easy to concentrate on the mortality and miss the important aspects of morbidity. However, outcome measures, and the relevant time to their measurement, may be guided by the studies themselves and not by your original question. This is particularly true, for example, when looking at pain relief, where the patient's objective may be "relief of pain" while the studies may define and assess this using a range of different measures.[1]

Type of question

Once you have created a question, it is helpful to think about what type of question you are asking, as this will affect where you look for the answer and what type of research you can expect to provide the answer.

Typology for question building

1. **Clinical findings**: how to interpret findings from the history and clinical examination.
2. **Aetiology**: the causes of disease and their modes of operation.
3. **Differential diagnosis**: when considering the possible causes of a patient's clinical problem, how to rank them by likelihood, seriousness and treatability.
4. **Prognosis:** the probable course of disease over time and prediction of likely outcomes.
5. **Therapy:** selection of treatments based on efficacy, cost and your patient's values.
6. **Prevention:** identifying primary and secondary risk factors, leading to therapy or behavioural change.
7. **Cost-effectiveness**: is one intervention more cost-effective than another?
8. **Quality of life**: what will be the quality of life of the patient following (or without) this intervention?

Consult the Levels of Evidence table on p50–4 to see what type of study would give you the best evidence for each type of question.

Deciding which question to ask

- Which question is most important to the patient's wellbeing? (Have you taken into account the patient's perspective?)
- Which question is most feasible to answer in the time you have available?
- Which question is most likely to benefit your clinical practice?
- Which question is most interesting to you?

Further reading

Educational Prescriptions: http://cebm.jr2.ox.ac.uk/docs/eduscrip.html

Gray J. Doing the Right Things Right. In: *Evidence Based Health-Care*. New York: Churchill Livingstone, 1997, chapter 2.

Richardson W, Wilson M, Nishikawa J, Hayward RS. The well-built clinical question: a key to evidence-based decisions [editorial]. *ACP J Club* 1995;**123**:A12–13. See also http://cebm.jr2. ox.ac.uk/docs/focusquest.html

Finding the evidence

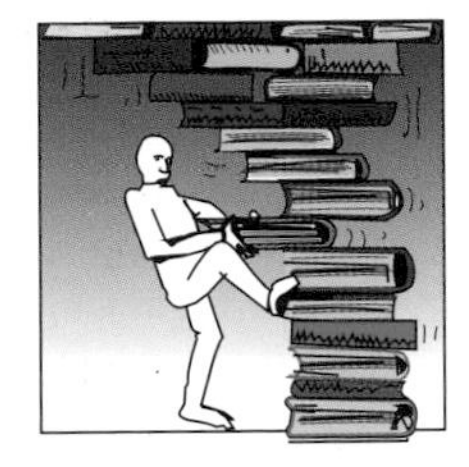

Convert your question to a search strategy

Identify terms which you would want to include in your search.

Patient or Problem	Intervention	Comparison	Outcome

Identify sources of evidence

1. Levels of evidence (see p50–4): what type of study would give you the best quality evidence for your question?
2. Critically Appraised Topics (see p57–61): is there a CAT available on your clinical question?
3. Secondary sources: is there a quality and relevance-filtered summary of evidence on your question, such as in *ACP Journal Club* or *Best Evidence*?
4. Systematic reviews: Is there a systematic review in the *Cochrane Library*?
5. Bibliographic databases: in which database would you find a relevant clinical trial?

Electronic sources of evidence

Source	*Availability*	*Advantages*	*Disadvantages*
CATs (see p57)	http://cebm.jr2.ox.ac.uk your collection	Pre-appraised summaries for a clinical question	Only one study per CAT; time-limited; quality control
Best Evidence	CD Rom	Pre-appraised summaries filtered for clinical relevance	Limited coverage
Cochrane Library	CD Rom, online from http://www.update-software.com	High-quality systematic reviews which cover a complete topic	Limited coverage, time lag, can be difficult to use
Bibliographic databases (MEDLINE, CINAHL, etc)	CD Rom, online	Original research articles, up-to-date	Difficult to search effectively, no quality filtering, bibliographic text

Secondary sources

Of course, if someone has already searched for and appraised evidence around your question, it makes sense to share that information if possible. One way this can be done, either for your own private use or for sharing with others, is in the form of Critically Appraised Topics or CATs. Many people make their CATs available on the web (see p57) and you might like to start searching here. You should be wary, however, of the provenance of these CATs: is there an explicit quality control process which has been applied to them and have they been updated recently?

Source	*http://*	*Contains*
Bandolier	www.jr2.ox.ac.uk/ Bandolier	User-friendly, searchable collection of evidence-based summaries and commentaries
TRIP	www.tripdatabase.com	Searchable database of links to evidence-based summaries and guidelines on the web

Secondary journals, such as *ACP Journal Club* and *Evidence-Based Medicine*, publish structured abstracts which summarise the best quality and most clinically useful recent research from the literature. This is an excellent way to use the limited time at your disposal for reading, and the Best Evidence CD Rom provides quick access to the back catalogue of both of these journals.

The Cochrane Library, which contains the full text of over 1000 systematic reviews, may be your next port of call. A good systematic review will summarise all of the high-quality published (and unpublished) research around a specific question. However, bear in mind that there may not be a systematic review which tackles your specific question, interpreting reviews can be time-consuming, and there may be more recent research which has not yet been incorporated into the review.

Choosing the right bibliographic database(s)

A bibliographic database consists of bibliographic records (usually with abstract) of published literature from journals, monographs, and serials. It is important to be aware that different bibliographic databases cover different subject areas, and to search the one(s) most relevant to your needs.

Database	Coverage
CINAHL	Nursing and allied health, health education, occupational and physiotherapy, social services
EMBASE	European equivalent of MEDLINE, with emphasis on drugs and pharmacology
MEDLINE	US database covering all aspects of clinical medicine, biological sciences, education, technology, and health-related social and information sciences
PsycLIT	Psychology, psychiatry and related disciplines, including sociology, linguistics and education

Search strategies for MEDLINE and other bibliographic databases

There are two main types of strategy for searching bibliographic databases: *thesaurus searching* (all articles are indexed under subject headings, so if you search for a specific heading you will pick up lots of potentially relevant materials) and *textword searching* (where you search for the occurrence of specific words or phrases in the article's bibliographic record).

*Unfortunately, the index may not correspond **exactly** to your needs (and the indexers may not have been consistent in the way they assigned articles to subject headings); similarly, using textword searching alone may miss important articles. For these reasons, you should use **both** thesaurus and textword searching where possible.*

Most databases allow you to build up a query by typing multiple statements which you can combine using Boolean operators (see below). Here is an example:

Question: In postmenopausal women, what are the effects of HRT on osteoporosis?

Textword search

#1 hormone OR ?estrogen
#2 #1AND therap*
#3 #2 OR HRT
#4 bone AND density
#5 #4 OR osteoporosis
#6 #3 AND #5

Thesaurus search

#1 Estrogen-Replacement Therapy/all subheadings
#2 Bone Density/all subheadings
#3 Osteoporosis/all subheadings
#4 #2 OR #3
#5 #1 AND #4

It is best to start your search by casting your net wide with both textword and thesaurus searching (a high-sensitivity search, to catch all the articles which may be relevant), and progressively narrowing it to exclude irrelevant items (increasing specificity).

To increase **sensitivity**:

1. Expand your search using (broader terms in) the *thesaurus*.
2. Use a *textword* search of the database.
3. Use *truncation* and *wildcards* to catch spelling variants.
4. Use *Boolean* OR to make sure you have included all alternatives for the terms you are after (for example (myocardial AND infarction) OR (heart AND attack)).

To increase **specificity**:

1. Use a *thesaurus* to identify more specific headings.
2. Use more specific terms in *textword* search.
3. Use *Boolean* AND to represent other aspects of the question.
4. *Limit* the search by publication type, year of publication, etc.

Depending on which databases you use, these features might have different keystrokes or commands associated with them; however, we have tried to summarise them as best we can in the table below.

Feature	*Key*	*Explanation*
Expand	thesaurus (MeSH)	Use *explosion* and *include all sub-headings* to expand your search.
Truncation	*(or $)	analy* = analysis, analytic, analytical, analyse, etc.
Wildcards	?	gyn?ecology = gynaecology, gynecology; randomi?* = randomisation, randomization, randomised.
Boolean	AND	Article must include both terms.
	OR	Article can include either term.
	NOT	Excludes articles containing the term (for example econom* NOT economy picks up economic and economical but not economy).
Proximity	NEAR	Terms must occur close to each other (for example within 6 words) (heart NEAR failure)
Limit	variable	As appropriate, restrict by publication type (clinical-trial.pt), year, language, possibly by study characteristics, or by searching for terms in specific parts of the document (for example diabet* in ti will search for articles which have diabetes or diabetic in the title).
Related	variable	Once you've found a useful article, this feature (for example in PubMed by clicking the "Related" hyperlink) searches for similar items in the database.

If you want to target high-quality evidence, it is possible to construct search strategies that will only pick up the best evidence; see the CASPfew web site for examples (http://wwwlib.jr2.ox.ac.uk/caspfew/filters/index.html). Some MEDLINE services provide such search "filters" online, so that you can click them or upload them automatically. However, you might also like to check out the **Levels of Evidence** on p50–4 to get an idea of what type of research would yield the best quality of information for each type of question (therapy, diagnosis, prognosis, etc.).

PubMed: MEDLINE on the internet

The US National Library of Medicine now offers its MEDLINE database free on the web at http://www3.ncbi.nlm.nih.gov/PubMed/. Here are some quick hints to help you to get the most out of this excellent service.

- Type search terms into the query box and click GO.
- Multiple terms are automatically ANDed unless you specifically include Boolean operators in UPPER CASE, for example (hormone replacement) OR hrt.
- Search terms are automatically truncated and mapped to the thesaurus.
- You can bypass truncation by enclosing your terms in double quotes.
- You can target a specific field of the record by following your query with the field code in square brackets: bloggs j [au] will search for *bloggs j* in the author field.
- Use the asterisk (*) for truncation
- The Details button allows you to view your search as PubMed translated it and to save your search (as a Bookmark in your browser).
- Once you've found a good article, use Related Articles to search for similar ones.

Consult PubMed's online help for more details.

Searching the internet

You might like to begin searching the internet using a specialised search engine which focuses on evidence-based sources. Two such services are TRIP (see above) and SUMSearch (http://sumsearch.uthscsa.edu/searchform45.htm) which searches other websites for you, optimising your search by question type and number of hits.

Generic internet search engines offer two main types of search: by category (where the search engine has classified web pages into subject category) or by free text search (where any occurrence of a term in a web page provides you with a "hit"). Obviously, the former strategy offers greater specificity, while the latter offers better sensitivity.

In searching for clinical information on the internet, you should be wary of the provenance of the material; ask yourself first: does this website have a clear quality control policy which has been applied to the material?

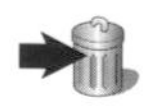

Using Yahoo! (www.yahoo.com)

Yahoo has a clear selection of categories, but there is considerable overlap between them, so it is worth doing a text search, which will list all the Yahoo categories as well as individual websites.

Feature	*Key*	*Explanation*
Truncation	*	analy* = analysis, analytic, analytical, analyse, etc.
Adjacency	" "	Words must be adjacent to each other: for example "heart attack"
AND	+	+natural +childbirth = documents must contain both words
Limits	t: u:	Words must occur in title of the document (t:natural childbirth) or words must occur in web address (u:uk)

Yahoo ranks the outcome of your search: documents that contain multiple matches with your search text are ranked highest; those that match your search in the document title are next highest. Other good search engines include Google (www.google.com), which has no advertising on its simple front-end and a very user-friendly search optimisation page.

Further reading

CASPfew: http://wwwlib.jr2.ox.ac.uk/caspfew/: includes introductory exercises, toolkit and sources guide.

CEBM: http:cebm.jr2.ox.ac.uk/docs/searching.html: includes tips on how to target high-quality trials on specific question types (therapy, diagnosis, etc.).

McKibbon A *et al. PDQ Evidence-Based Principles and Practice*. Hamilton, ON: BC Decker, 2000.

Snowball R. Finding the evidence: an information skills approach. In M Dawes (ed.), *Evidence-based Practice: a primer for health care professionals*. Edinburgh: Churchill Livingstone, 1999, pp15–46.

The SCHARR guide to EBP on the internet: http://www.shef.ac.uk/~scharr/ir/netting.html.

Appraising therapy articles

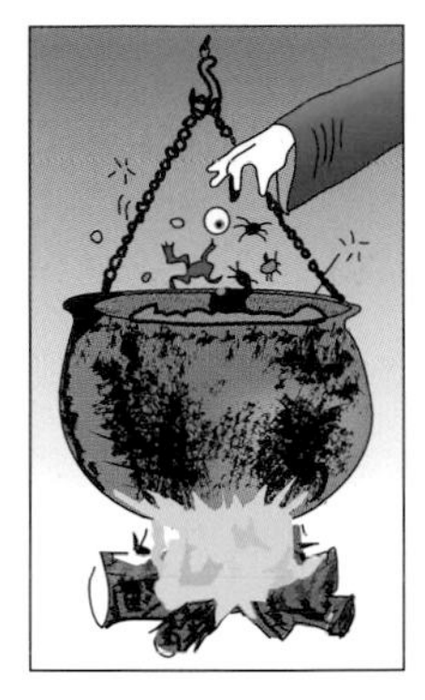

Is the study valid?

1. Was there a clearly defined research question?
2. Was the assignment of patients to treatments randomised and was the randomisation list concealed?
3. Were all patients accounted for at its conclusion? Was there an "intention-to-treat" analysis?
4. Were research participants "blinded"?
5. Were the groups treated equally throughout?
6. Did randomisation produce comparable groups at the start of the trial?

Are the results important?

Relative Risk Reduction (RRR) = (CER − EER) / CER
Absolute Risk Reduction (ARR) = CER − EER
Number Needed to Treat (NNT) = 1 / ARR

Is the study valid?

1. Was there a clearly defined research question?

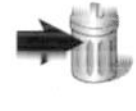

What question has the research been designed to answer? Was the question focused in terms of the population group studied, the intervention received and the outcomes considered?

2. Were the groups randomised?

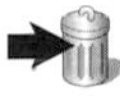

The most important type of research for answering therapy questions is the randomised controlled trial (RCT). The major reason for randomisation is to create two (or more) comparison groups which are similar. To reduce bias as much as possible, the decision as to which treatment a patient receives should be determined by random allocation.

Concealed randomisation

As a supplementary point, clinicians who are entering patients into a trial may consciously or unconsciously distort the balance between groups if they know the treatments given to previous patients. For this reason, it is preferable that the randomisation list be concealed from the clinicians.

> ***Why is this important?***
> *Randomisation is important because it spreads all confounding variables evenly amongst the study groups, even the ones we don't know about.*

Stratified randomisation

True random allocation can result in some differences occurring between the two groups through chance, particularly if the sample size is small. This can lead to difficulty when analysing the results if, for instance, there was an important difference in severity of disease between the two groups. Using stratified randomisation, the researcher identifies the most important factors relevant to that research question; randomisation is then stratified such that these factors are equally distributed in the control and experimental groups.

3. Were all patients accounted for at its conclusion?

There are three major aspects to assessing the follow up of trials:

- Did so many patients drop out of the trial that its results are in doubt?
- Was the study long enough to allow outcomes to become manifest?
- Were patients analysed in the groups to which they were originally assigned (intention-to-treat)?

Drop-out rates

The undertaking of a clinical trial is usually time-consuming and difficult to complete properly. If less than 80% of patients are adequately followed up then the results may be invalid. The American College of Physicians has decided to use 80% as its threshold for inclusion of papers into the *ACP Journal* and *Evidence-Based Medicine*.

Length of study

Studies must allow enough time for outcomes to become manifest. You should use your clinical judgement to decide whether this was true for the study you are appraising, and whether the length of follow up was appropriate to the outcomes you are interested in.

Intention-to-treat

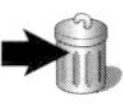

Sometimes, patients may change treatment aims during the course of a study, for all sorts of reasons. If we analysed the patients on the basis of what treatment they got rather than what they were allocated (intention-to-treat), we have altered the even distribution of confounders produced by randomisation. So, all patients should be analysed in the groups to which they were originally randomised, even if this is not the treatment they actually got.

4. Were the research participants "blinded"?

Ideally, patients and clinicians should not know whether they are receiving the treatment. The assessors may unconsciously bias their assessment of outcomes if they are aware of the treatment. This is known as observer bias.

So, the ideal trial would blind patients, carers, assessors and analysts alike. The terms single, double and triple blind are sometimes used to describe these permutations. However, there is some variation in their usage and you should check to see exactly who was blinded in a trial. Of course, it may have been impossible to blind certain groups of participants, depending on the type of intervention. Note also that concealment of randomisation, which happens before patients are enrolled, is different from blinding, which happens afterwards.

Placebo control

Patients do better if they think they are receiving a treatment than if they do not; the placebo effect is a widely accepted potential bias in trials.

So, the ideal trial would perform **"double-blind" randomisation** (where both the patient and the clinician do not know whether they are receiving active or placebo treatment), and where the randomisation list is concealed from the clinician allocating treatment (see above). In some cases, it would not be possible to blind either or both of the participants (depending on the type of intervention and outcome), but researchers should endeavour to carry out blind allocation and assessment of outcomes wherever possible.

5. Equal treatment

It should be clear from the article that, for example, there were no co-interventions which were applied to one group but not the other and that the groups were followed similarly with similar check-ups.

6. Did randomisation produce comparable groups at the start of the trial?

The purpose of randomisation is to generate two (or more) groups of patients who are similar in all important ways. The authors should allow you to check this by displaying important characteristics of the groups in tabular form.

Outcome measures

An outcome measure is any feature that is recorded to determine the progression of the disease or problem being studied. Outcomes should be objectively defined and measured wherever possible. Often, outcomes are expressed as mean values of measures rather than numbers of individuals having a particular outcome. The use of means can hide important information about the characteristics of patients who have improved and, perhaps more importantly, those who have got worse.

Are the results important?

Two things you need to consider are how large is the treatment effect and how precise is the finding from the trial.

In any clinical therapeutic study there are three explanations for the observed effect:

1. Bias.
2. Chance variation between the two groups.
3. The effect of the treatment.

Once bias has been excluded (by asking if the study is valid), we must consider the possibility that the results are a chance effect.

p Values

Alongside the results, the paper should report a measure of the likelihood that this result could have occurred if the treatment was no better than the control. The *p* value is a commonly used measure of this probability.

For example, a p value of <0.01 means that there is a less than 1 in 100 (1%) probability of the result occurring by chance; $p<0.05$ means this is less than 1 in 20 probability.

Quantifying the risk of benefit and harm

Once chance and bias have been ruled out, we must examine the difference in event rates between the control and experimental groups to see if there is a significant difference. These **event rates** can be calculated as shown below:

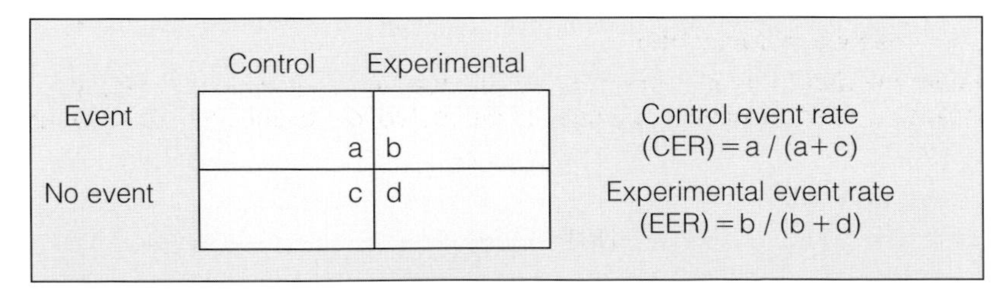

	Control	Experimental
Event	a	b
No event	c	d

Control event rate (CER) = a / (a+c)

Experimental event rate (EER) = b / (b + d)

Relative risk reduction (RRR)

Relative risk reduction is the percentage reduction in events in the treated group event rate (EER) compared to the control group event rate (CER):

$$RRR = \frac{CER - EER}{CER}$$

Absolute risk reduction (ARR)

Absolute risk reduction is the absolute difference between the control and experimental group.

$$ARR = CER - EER$$

ARR is a more clinically relevant measure to use than RRR. This is because RRR "factors out" the baseline risk, so that small differences in risk can seem significant when compared to a small baseline risk. Consider the two sets of sample figures below, where the same RRR is found even though the treatment shows ten times greater absolute benefit in sample 1:

	CER	EER	ARR	RRR
1	0.36 (36%)	0.34 (34%)	0.36 − 0.34 = 0.02 (2%)	(0.36 − 0.34) / 0.36 = 5.6%
2	0.036% (3.6%)	0.034 (3.4%)	0.036 − 0.034 = 0.002 (0.2%)	(0.036 − 0.034) / 0.036 = 5.6%

Number needed to treat (NNT)

Number needed to treat is the most useful measure of benefit, as it tells you the absolute number of patients who need to be treated to prevent one bad outcome. It is the inverse of the ARR:

$$NNT = \frac{1}{ARR}$$

Mortality in patients surviving acute myocardial infarction for at least 3 days with left ventricular ejection fraction <40% (ISIS-4, *Lancet* 1995)		Relative risk reduction (RRR)	Absolute risk reduction (ARR)	Number needed to treat (NNT)
Placebo: control event rate (CER)	Captopril: experimental event rate (EER)	$\frac{CER - EER}{CER}$	CER − EER	**1 / ARR**
275 / 1116 = 0.2464 (24.64%)	228 / 1115 = 0.2045 (20.45%)	$\frac{0.2464 - 0.2045}{0.2464}$ = 17%	0.2464 − 0.2054 = 0.0419 (4.19%)	**1 / 0.0419 = 24** (NNTs always round UP)

Confidence intervals (CIs)

Any study can only examine a sample of a population. Hence, we would expect the sample to be different from the population. This is known as *sampling error*. Confidence intervals (CIs) are used to represent sampling error. A 95% CI specifies that there is a 95% chance that the population's "true" value lies between the two limits. The 95% CI on an NNT = 1 / the 95% CI on its ARR:

$$\text{95\% CI on the ARR} = \pm/1.96 \times \sqrt{\frac{CER \times (1 - CER)}{\text{\# of control patients}} + \frac{EER \times (1 - EER)}{\text{\# of exper. patients}}}$$

If a confidence interval crosses the "line of no difference" (i.e. the point at which a benefit becomes a harm), then we can conclude that the results are *not statistically significant*.

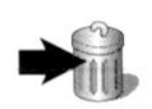

Relative risk (RR)

Relative risk is also used to quantify the difference in risk between control and experimental groups. Relative risk is a ratio of the risk in the experimental group to the risk in the control group.

$$RR = EER / CER$$

Thus, an RR below 1 shows that there is less risk of the event in the experimental group. As with the RRR, relative risk does not tell you anything about the baseline risk, or therefore the absolute benefit to be gained.

Summary

An evidence-based approach to deciding whether a treatment is effective for your patient involves the following steps:

1. Frame the clinical question.
2. Search for evidence concerning the efficacy of the therapy.
3. Assess the methods used to carry out the trial of the therapy.
4. Determine the NNT of the therapy.
5. Decide whether the NNT can apply to your patient, and estimate a particularised NNT.
6. Incorporate your patient's values and preferences into deciding on a course of action.

Further reading

Bandolier Guide to Bias: http://www.jr2.ox.ac.uk/bandolier/band80/b80-2.html

Dawes M *et al. Evidence-Based Practice: a primer for health care professionals.* Edinburgh: Churchill Livingstone, 1999, pp. 49–58.

Greenhalgh P. *How to Read a Paper, 2nd ed.* London: BMJ Books, 2001.

Guyatt GH *et al.* Users' Guides to the Medical Literature II: How to use an article about therapy or prevention A: Are the results of the study valid? *JAMA* 1993;**270**(21):2598–601.

Guyatt GH *et al.* Users' Guides to the Medical Literature II: How to use an article about therapy or prevention B: What were the results and will they help me in caring for my patients? *JAMA* 1994:**271**(1):59–63.

ISIS-4 (Fourth International Study of Infarct Survival) Collaborative Group. *Lancet* 1995:**345**:669–85. See also the CAT at www.eboncall.co.uk

Sackett DL *et al. Evidence-Based Medicine: How to practice and teach EBM.* New York: Churchill Livingstone, 2000.

Appraising diagnosis articles

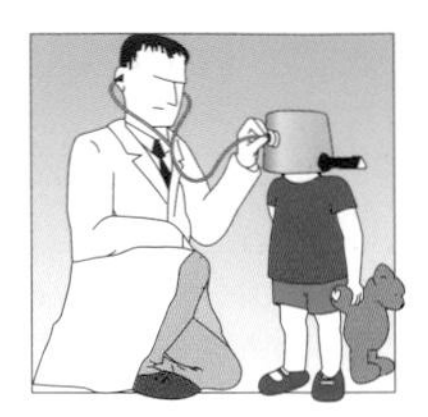

Is the study valid?

1. Was there a clearly defined question?
2. Was the presence or absence of the target disorder confirmed with a validated test ("gold" or reference standard)?
   - Was this comparison independent from and blind to the study test results?
3. Was the test evaluated on an appropriate spectrum of patients?
4. Was the reference standard applied to all patients?

Are the results important?

		Target Disorder		
		Present	Absent	Totals
Test result	Positive	a	b	a+b
	Negative	c	d	c+d
	Totals	a+c	b+d	a+b+c+d

Sensitivity = a/(a+c) =

Specificity = d/(b+d) =

Likelihood ratio for a positive test result = LR + = sens/(1 − spec) =

Likelihood ratio for a negative test result = LR− = (1 − sens)/spec =

Is the study valid?

1. Was there a clearly defined question?

What question has the research been designed to answer? Was the question focused in terms of the population group studied, the target disorder and the test(s) considered?

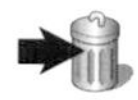

2. Was the presence or absence of the target disorder confirmed with a validated test ("gold" or reference standard)?

How did the investigators know whether or not a patient in the study really had the disease? To do this, they will have needed some reference standard test (or series of tests) which they know "always" tells the truth. You need to consider whether the reference standard used is sufficiently accurate.

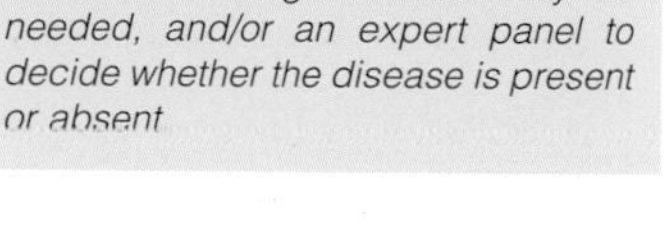

Sometimes, there may not be a single test that is suitable as a reference standard. A range of tests may be needed, and/or an expert panel to decide whether the disease is present or absent.

Were the reference standard and the diagnostic test interpreted blind and independently of each other?

If the study investigators know the result of the reference standard test, this might influence their interpretation of the diagnostic test and vice versa.

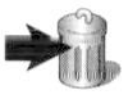

3. Was the test evaluated on an appropriate spectrum of patients?

A test may perform differently depending upon the sort of patients on whom it is carried out. A test is going to perform better in terms of detecting people with disease if it is used on people in whom the disease is more severe or advanced. Similarly, the test will produce more false positive results if it is carried out on patients with other diseases that might mimic the disease that is being tested for. The issue to consider when appraising a paper is whether the test was evaluated on the typical sort of patients on whom the test would be carried out in real life.

4. Was the reference standard applied to all patients?

Ideally, both the test being evaluated and the reference standard should be carried out on all patients in the study. For example, if the test under investigation proves positive, there may be a temptation not to bother administering the reference standard test. Therefore, when reading the paper you need

However, this may not be possible for both practical and ethical reasons. For example, the reference test may be invasive and may expose the patient to some risk and/or discomfort.

to find out whether the reference standard was applied to all patients, and if it wasn't look at what steps the investigators took to find out what the "truth" was in patients who did not have the reference test.

Is it clear how the test was carried out?

To be able to apply the results of the study to your own clinical practice, you need to be confident that the test is performed in the same way in your setting as it was in the study.

Is the test result reproducible?

This is essentially asking whether you get the same result if different people carry out the test, or if the test is carried out at different times on the same person. Many studies will assess this by having different observers perform the test, and measuring the agreement between them by means of a kappa statistic. The **kappa** statistic takes into account the amount of agreement that you would expect by chance.

For example, if two observers made a diagnosis by tossing a coin, you would expect them to agree 50% of the time. A kappa score of 0 indicates no more agreement than you would expect by chance; perfect agreement would yield a kappa score of 1. Generally, a kappa score of 0.6 indicates good agreement.

If agreement between observers is poor, then this will undermine the usefulness of the test. The extent to which the test result is reproducible or not may to some extent depend upon how explicit the guidance is for how the test should be carried out. It may also depend upon the experience and expertise of the observer.

Are the results important?

What is meant by test accuracy?

(a) The test can correctly detect disease that is present (a true positive result).
(b) The test can detect disease when it is really absent (a false positive result).
(c) The test can identify someone as being free of a disease when it is really present (a false negative result).
(d) The test can correctly identify that someone does not have a disease (a true negative result).

Ideally, we would like a test which produces a high proportion of (a) and (d) and a low proportion of (b) and (c).

- **Sensitivity**: is the proportion of people with disease who have a positive test.
- **Specificity**: is the proportion of people free of a disease who have a negative test.

These measures are combined into an overall measure of the efficacy of a diagnostic test called the **likelihood ratio**: the likelihood that a given test result would be expected in a patient with the target disorder compared to the likelihood that the same result would be expected in a patient without the disorder (see p39).

These possible outcomes of a diagnostic test are illustrated below[1] (sample data from Anriole *et al*.).

		Target disorder (prostate cancer)		Totals
		Present	Absent	
Diagnostic test result (prostate serum antigen)	Positive (<65 mmol/l)	26 **a**	**b** 69	95 **a+b**
	Negative (>65 mmol/l)	**c** 46	**d** 249	**c+d** 295
	Totals	**a+c** 72	**b+d** 318	**a+b+c+d** 390

Sensitivity = a/(a + c)	26/72	=36%
Specificity = d/(b + d)	249/318	=78%
Positive predictive value = a/(a + b)	26/95	=27%
Negative predictive value = d/(c + d)	249/295	=84%
Pre-test probability (prevalence) = (a + c)/(a + b + c + d)	72/390	=18%
Likelihood ratio for a **positive** test result = sens/(1 − spec)	0.36/0.22	=1.66
Likelihood ratio for a **negative** test result = (1 − sens)/spec	0.64/0.78	=0.82
Pre-test odds = prevalence/(1 − prevalence)	0.18/0.82	=0.22
For a positive test result:		
Post-test odds = pre-test odds × likelihood ratio	0.22 × 1.66	=0.37
Post-test probability = post-test odds/(post-test odds + 1)	0.37/1.37	=27%

Using sensitivity and specificity: SpPin and SnNout

Sometimes it can be helpful just knowing the sensitivity and specificity of a test, if they are very high. If a test has high specificity, i.e. if a high proportion of patients without the disorder actually test negative, it is unlikely to produce false positive results. Therefore, if the test is positive it makes the diagnosis very

Sensitivity reflects how good the test is at picking up people with disease, while the specificity reflects how good the test is at identifying people without the disease.

likely. This can be remembered by the mnemonic **SpPin**: for a test with high specificity (Sp), if the test is Positive, then it rules the diagnosis "in". Similarly, with high sensitivity a test is unlikely to produce false negative results. This can be remembered by the mnemonic **SnNout**: for a test with high sensitivity (Sn), if the test is Negative, then it rules "out" the diagnosis.

Effect of prevalence on predictive value

Positive predictive value is the percentage of patients who test positive who actually have the disease. Predictive values are affected by the prevalence of the disease: if a disease is rarer, the positive predictive value will be lower, while sensitivity and specificity are constant. Since we know that prevalence changes in different health care settings, predictive values are not generally very useful in characterising the accuracy of tests.

The measure of test accuracy that is most useful when it comes to interpreting test results for individual patients is the **likelihood ratio (LR)**. The next section shows how the LR can be used to derive a probability that the patient has the disease given a particular test result.

Summary

1. Frame the clinical question.
2. Search for evidence concerning the accuracy of the test.
3. Assess the methods used to determine the accuracy of the test.
4. Find out the likelihood ratios for the test.
5. Estimate the pre-test probability of disease in your patient.
6. Apply the likelihood ratios to this pre-test probability using the nomogram to determine what the post-test probability would be for different possible test results.
7. Decide whether or not to perform the test on the basis of your assessment of whether it will influence the care of the patient, and the patient's attitude to different possible outcomes.

References

1. Anriole GL *et al.* Treatment with finasteride preserves usefulness of prostate-specific antigen in the detection of prostate cancer: results of a randomised, double-blind, placebo-controlled clinical trial. *Urology* 1998;**52**(2):195–202.
2. Altman D. *Practical Statistics for Medical Research.* Edinburgh: Churchill Livingstone, 1991.
3. Fagan TJ. A nomogram for Bayes' Theorem. N *Engl J Med* 1975;**293**:257.
4. Sackett DL *et al. Evidence-Based Medicine: How to practice and teach EBM.* New York: Churchill Livingstone, 2000.

Further reading

Fleming KA. Evidence-based pathology. *Evidence-Based Medicine* 1997;**2**:132.

Jaeschke R *et al.* Users' Guides to the Medical Literature III: How to use an article about a diagnostic test A: Are the results of the study valid? *JAMA* 1994;**271**(5):389–91.

Jaeschke R *et al.* How to use an article about a diagnostic test A: What are the results and will they help me in caring for my patients? *JAMA* 1994;**271**(9):703–7.

Mant J. Studies assessing diagnostic tests. In: M Dawes *et al. Evidence-Based Practice: a primer for health care professionals.* Edinburgh: Churchill Livingstone, 1999, pp59–67,133–57.

Richardson WS, Wilson MC, Guyatt GH, Cook DJ, Nishikawa J. How to use an article about disease probability for differential diagnosis. *JAMA* 1999;**281**:1214–19.

Sackett DL, Haynes RB, Guyatt GH, Tugwell P. *Clinical epidemiology; a basic science for clinical medicine*, 2nd ed. Boston: Little, Brown, 1991.

Nomogram for likelihood ratios

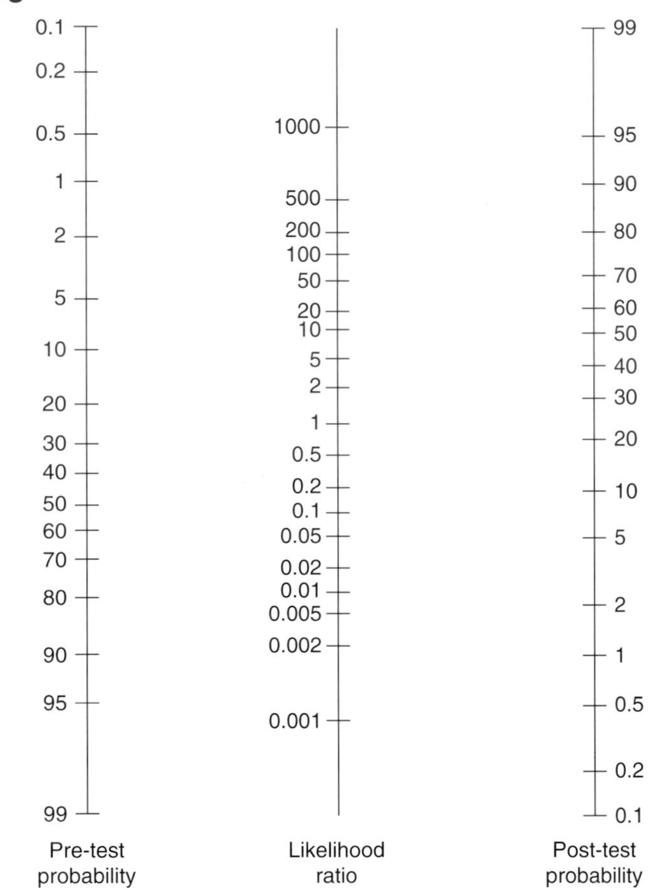

How to use the nomogram[3,4]

Position a ruler (or any straight edge) so that it connects the point on the left hand scale which corresponds to your (estimate of your) patient's pre-test probability with the point on the middle scale for the likelihood ratio for their test result. Now read off the post-test probability on the right-hand scale.

http://cebm.jr2.ox.ac.uk/docs/nomogram.html

Appraising systematic reviews

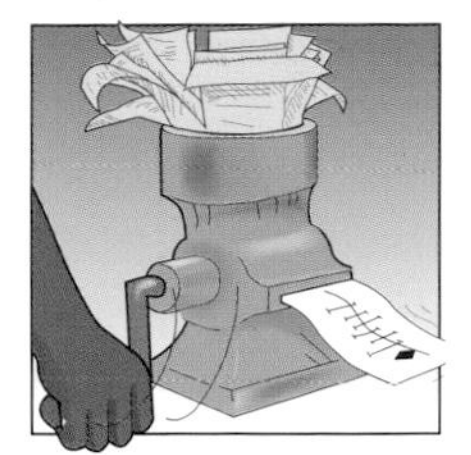

Is the systematic review valid?

1. Is it a systematic review of high-quality studies which are relevant to your question?
2. Does the methods section adequately describe:
   - a comprehensive search for all the relevant studies?
   - how the reviewers assessed the validity of each study?
3. Are the studies consistent, both clinically and statistically?

Are the results important?

If the review reports odds ratios (ORs), you can generate an NNT if you have an estimate of your patient's expected event rate (PEER).

$$NNT = \frac{1 - \{PEER \times (1 - OR)\}}{(1 - PEER) \times PEER \times (1 - OR)}$$

A systematic review is "a review of a clearly formulated question that uses systematic and explicit methods to identify, select and critically appraise relevant research, and to collect and analyse data from studies that are included in the review. Statistical methods may or may not be used to analyse and summarise the results of the included studies" (Cochrane Library 1998, Glossary).

Three key features of such a review are:
- a strenuous effort to locate all original reports on the topic of interest
- critical evaluation of the reports
- conclusions are drawn based on a synthesis of studies which meet pre-set quality criteria

When synthesising results, a meta-analysis may be undertaken. This is "the use of statistical techniques in a systematic review to integrate the results of the included studies" (Cochrane Library 1998, Glossary), which means that the authors have attempted to synthesise the different results into one overall statistic. The best source of systematic reviews is the Cochrane Library, available by subscription on CD or via the internet. Many of the systematic reviews so far completed are based on evidence of effectiveness of an intervention from randomised controlled trials (RCTs).

Is the systematic review valid?

1. Is it a systematic review of high-quality studies which are relevant to your question?

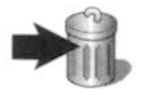

This question asks whether the research question in the review is clearly defined and the same as the one you are considering, and whether the studies covered by the review are high quality. Reviews of poor-quality studies simply compound the problems of poor-quality individual studies. Sometimes, reviews combine the results of variable-quality trials (for example randomised and non-randomised trials in therapy); the authors should provide separate information on the subset of randomised trials.

2. Does the methods section describe how all the relevant trials were found and assessed?

The paper should give a comprehensive account of the sources consulted in the search for relevant papers, the search strategy used to find them, **and** the quality and relevance criteria used to decide whether to include them in the review.

> *The reviewers' search should aim to minimise* ***publication bias:*** *the tendency for negative results to be unequally reported in the literature.*

Search strategy

Some questions you can ask about the search strategy:

- The authors should include hand searching of journals and searching for unpublished literature.
- Were any obvious databases missed?
- Did the authors check the reference lists of articles and of textbooks (citation indexing)?
- Did they contact experts (to get their list of references checked for completeness and to try and find out about ongoing or unpublished research)?
- Did they use an appropriate search strategy: were important subject terms missed?

Did the authors assess the trials' individual validity?

You should look for a statement of how the trials' validity was assessed. Ideally, two or more investigators should have applied these criteria independently and achieved good agreement in their results.

You need to know what criteria were used to select the research.

> *The importance of a clear statement of inclusion criteria is that studies should be selected on the basis of these criteria (that is, any study that matches these criteria is included) rather than selecting the study on the basis of the results.*

These should include who the study participants were, what was done to them, and what outcomes were assessed. A point to consider is that the narrower the inclusion criteria, the less generalisable are the results. However, this needs to be balanced with using very broad inclusion criteria, when heterogeneity (see below) becomes an issue.

3. Are the studies consistent, both clinically and statistically?

You have to use your clinical knowledge to decide whether the groups of patients, interventions, and outcome measures were similar enough to merit combining their results. If not, this **clinical heterogeneity** would invalidate the review.

Similarly, you would question the review's validity if the trials' results contradicted each other. Unless this **statistical heterogeneity** can be explained satisfactorily (such as by differences in patients, dosage, or durations of treatment), this should lead you to be very cautious about believing any overall conclusion from the review.

Are the results important?

Terms that you will probably come across when looking at systematic reviews include vote counting, odds ratios, and relative risks, amongst others.

Vote counting

If a systematic review does not contain a meta-analysis (a statistical method for combining the data from separate trials), the results may be presented as a simple count of the number of studies supporting an intervention and the number not supporting it. This assumes equal weight being given to each study, regardless of size.

Odds ratio (OR)

In measuring the efficacy of a therapy, odds can be used to describe risk. The odds of an event are the probability of it occurring compared to the probability of it not occurring.

By dividing the odds of an event in the experimental group by the odds in the control group, we can measure the efficacy of the treatment. ORs are useful because they can be used in a meta-analysis to combine the results of many different trials into one overall measure of efficacy.

If the experimental group has lower odds, the OR will be less than 1; if the control group has lower odds, the OR will be above 1; and if there is no difference between the two groups, the OR will be exactly 1.

To calculate the NNT for any OR and PEER:

$$NNT = \frac{1 - [PEER \times (1 - OR)]}{(1 - PEER) \times PEER \times (1 - OR)}$$

Logarithmic odds

Odds ratios are usually plotted on a log scale to give an equal line length on either side of the line of "no difference". If odds ratios are plotted on a log scale, then a log odds ratio of 0 means no effect, and whether or not the 95% confidence interval crosses a vertical line through zero will lead to a decision about its significance.

Binary or continuous data

Binary data (an event rate: something that either happens or not, such as numbers of patients improved or not) is usually combined using odds ratios. Continuous data (such as numbers of days, peak expiratory flow rate) is combined using differences in mean values for treatment and control groups (weighted mean differences or WMD) when units of measurement are the same, or standardised mean differences when units of measurement differ. Here the difference in means is divided by the pooled standard deviation.

How precise are the results?

The statistical significance of the results will depend on the extent of any confidence limits around the result (see p17). The review should include confidence intervals for all results, both of individual studies and any meta-analysis.

Further reading

Altman D. *Practical Statistics for Medical Research*. Edinburgh: Churchill Livingstone, 1991.

Antman EM, Lau J, Kupelnick B, Mosteller F, Chalmers TC. A comparison of results of meta-analyses of randomised control trials and recommendations of clinical experts. *JAMA* 1992;**268**:240–8.

Cochrane Library: http://www.update-software.com

NHS Centre for Reviews and Dissemination: http://www.york.ac.uk/inst/crd/

Oxman AD *et al.* Users' Guides to the Medical Literature VI: How to use an overview. *JAMA* 1994;**272**(17):1367–71.

Sackett DC, Straus SE, Richardson WS, Rosenberg W, Haynes RB. *Evidence-Based Medicine: How to practice and teach EBM*. Churchill Livingstone, 2000.

Seers K. Systematic review. In M Dawes *et al.* (eds) *Evidence-Based Practice: a primer for health care professionals*. Edinburgh: Churchill Livingstone, 1999, pp85–100.

Appraising articles on harm/aetiology

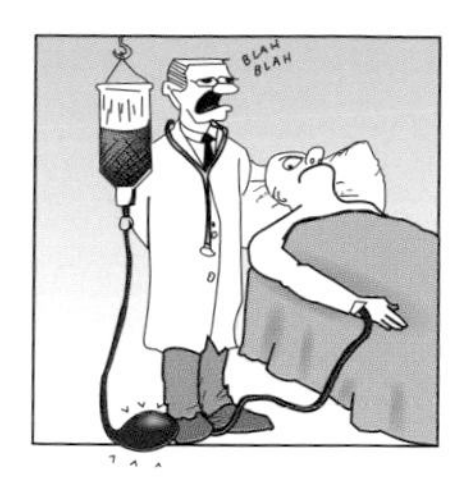

Is the study valid?

1. Was there a clearly defined research question?
2. Were there clearly defined, similar groups of patients?
3. Were exposures and clinical outcomes measured the same ways in both groups?
4. Was the follow up complete and long enough?
5. Does the suggested causative link make sense?

Are the valid results from this study important?

		Adverse outcome		
		Present (case)	Absent (control)	Totals
Exposure	Yes (Cohort)	a	b	a + b
	No (Cohort)	c	d	c + d
Totals		a + c	b + d	a + b + c + d

In a randomised trial or cohort study: **Relative risk** = RR = [a/(a+b)]/[c/(c + d)]

In a case–control study: Odds ratio = OR = ad/bc

Is the study valid?

In assessing an intervention's potential for harm, we are usually looking at prospective cohort studies or retrospective case–control studies. This is because RCTs may have to be very large indeed to pick up small adverse reactions to treatment.

1. Was there a clearly defined question?

What question has the research been designed to answer? Was the question focused in terms of the population group studied, the exposure received, and the outcomes considered?

2. Were there clearly defined, similar groups of patients?

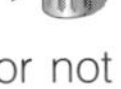

Studies looking at harm must be able to demonstrate that the two groups of patients are clearly defined and sufficiently similar so as to be comparable. In a cohort study, for example, patients are either exposed to the treatment or not according to a decision; this might mean that sicker patients, perhaps more likely to have adverse outcomes, are more likely to be offered (or demand) potentially helpful treatment. There may be some statistical adjustment to the results to take these potential confounders into account.

3. Were treatment exposures and clinical outcomes measured the same ways in both groups?

You would not want one group to be studied more exhaustively than the other, because this might lead to reporting a greater occurrence of exposure or outcome in the more intensively studied group.

4. Was the follow up complete and long enough?

Follow up has to be long enough for the harmful effects to reveal themselves, and complete enough for the results to be trustworthy (the 80% rule from p13 applies: lost patients may have very different outcomes from those who remain in the study).

5. Does the suggested causative link make sense?

You can apply the following rationale to help decide if the results make sense.

- ***Is it clear the exposure preceded the onset of the outcome?***

It must be clear that the exposure wasn't just a "marker" of another disease.

- ***Is there a dose–response gradient?***

If the exposure was causing the outcome, you might expect to see increased harmful effects as a result of increased exposure: a dose–response effect.

- ***Is there evidence from a "dechallenge–rechallenge" study?***

Does the adverse effect decrease when the treatment is withdrawn ("dechallenge") and worsen or reappear when the treatment is restarted ("rechallenge")?

- ***Is the association consistent from study to study?***

Try finding other studies, or, ideally, a systematic review of the question.

- ***Does the association make biological sense?***

If it does, a causal association is more likely.

Are the results important?

This means looking at the risk or odds of the adverse effect with (as opposed to without) exposure to the treatment; the higher the risk or odds, the stronger the association and the more we should be impressed by it. We can use the single table to determine if the valid results of the study are important.

		Adverse outcome		
		Present (case)	Absent (control)	Totals
Exposure	Yes (Cohort)	a	b	a + b
	No (Cohort)	c	d	c + d
Totals		a + c	b + d	a + b + c + d

In a cohort study: Relative risk = RR = [a/(a+b)]/[c/(c + d)]

In a case–control study: Odds ratio = OR = ad/bc

To calculate the NNH for any OR and PEER:

$$NNH = \frac{[PEER (OR - 1)] + 1}{PEER (OR - 1) \times (1 - PEER)}$$

A cohort study compares the risk of an adverse event amongst patients who received the exposure of interest with the risk in a similar group who did not receive it. Therefore, we are able to calculate a relative risk (or risk ratio) In case–control studies, we are presented with the outcomes, and work backwards looking at exposures. Here, we can only compare the two groups in terms of their relative odds (odds ratio).

Statistical significance

As with other measures of efficacy, we would be concerned if the 95% CI around the results, whether relative risk or odds ratio, crossed the value of 1, meaning that there may be no effect (or the opposite).

Further reading

Levine M *et al.* Users' Guides to the Medical Literature IV: How to use an article about harm. *JAMA* 1994;**272**(20): 1615-19.

Sackett DL, Haynes RB, Guyatt GH, Tugwell P. *Clinical epidemiology. A basic science for clinical medicine*, 2nd ed. Boston: Little, Brown, 1991.

Sackett DL *et al. Evidence-Based Medicine: How to practice and teach EBM.* New York: Churchill Livingstone, 1996.

Appraising prognosis studies

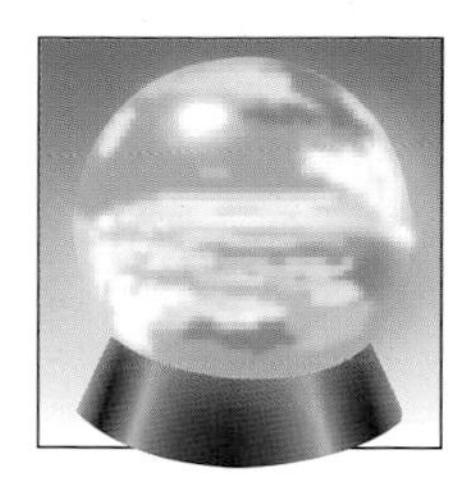

Is the sample representative?

Were they recruited at a common point in their illness?

Did the study account for other important factors?

Is the setting representative?

Was follow up long enough for the clinical outcome?

Was follow up complete?

Were outcomes measured "blind"?

Are the results important?

What is the risk of the outcome over time?

How precise are the estimates?

95% Confidence Intervals are ± 1.96 times the Standard Error (SE) of the measure.
SE of a proportion;

$$SE = \sqrt{\frac{p \times (1-p)}{n}}$$

Is the study valid?

In asking questions about a patient's likely prognosis over time, the best individual study type to look for would be longitudinal cohort study.

Is the sample representative

Does the study clearly define the group of patients, and is it similar to your patients? Were there clear inclusion and exclusion criteria?

Were they recruited at a common point in their illness?

The methodology should include a clear description of the stage and timing of the illness being studied. To avoid missing outcomes, study patients should ideally be recruited at an early stage in the disease. In any case, they should all be recruited at a consistent stage in the disease; if not, this will bias the results.

Did the study account for other important factors?

The study groups will have different important variables such as sex, age, weight and co-morbidity which could affect their outcome. The investigators should adjust their analysis to take account of these known factors in different sub-groups of patients. You should use your clinical judgement to assess whether any important factors were left out of this analysis and whether the adjustments were appropriate. This information will also help you in deciding how this evidence applies to your patient.

Is the setting representative?

Patients who are referred to specialist centres often have more illnesses and are higher risk than those cared for in the community. This is sometimes called "referral bias".

Was follow up long enough for the clinical outcome?

You have to be sure that the study followed the patients for long enough for the outcomes to manifest themselves. Longer follow up may be necessary in chronic diseases.

Was follow up complete?

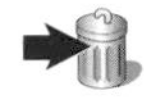

Most studies will lose some patients to follow up; the question you have to answer is whether so many were lost that the information is of no use to you.

You should look carefully in the paper for an account of why patients were lost and consider whether this introduces bias into the result.

- If follow up is less than 80% the study's validity is seriously undermined.

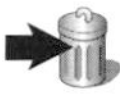

You can ask "what if" all those patients who were lost to follow up had the outcome you were interested in, and compare this with the study to see if loss to follow up had a significant effect. With low incidence conditions, loss to follow up is more problematic.

Were outcomes measured "blind"?

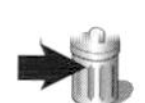

How did the study investigators tell whether or not the patients actually had the outcome? The investigators should have defined the outcome/s of interest in advance and have clear criteria which they used to determine whether the outcome had occurred. Ideally, these should be objective, but often some degree of interpretation and clinical judgement will be required. To eliminate potential bias in these situations, judgements should have been applied without knowing the patient's clinical characteristics and prognostic factors.

Are the results important?

What is the risk of the outcome over time?

Three ways in which outcomes might be presented are:

- as a percentage of survival at a particular point in time;
- as a median survival (the length of time by which 50% of study patients have had the outcome);
- as a survival curve that depicts, at each point in time, the proportion (expressed as a percentage) of the original study sample who have not yet had a specified outcome.

Survival curves provide the advantage that you can see how the patient's risk might develop over time.

How precise are the estimates?

Any study looks at a sample of the population, so we would expect some variation between the sample and "truth". Prognostic estimates should be accompanied by Confidence Intervals to represent this. A 95% Confidence Interval is the range of values between which we can be 95% sure that the true value lies. You should take account of this range when extracting estimates for your patient. If it is very wide, you would question whether the study had enough patients to provide useful information.

$$SE = \sqrt{\frac{p \times (1-p)}{n}}$$

Assuming a Normal distribution, the 95% Confidence Interval is 1.96 times this value on either side of the estimate.

Further Reading

Laupacis A, Wells G, Richardson WS, Tugwell P. Users' guides to the medical literature. V. How to use an article about prognosis. *JAMA* 1994;**272:**234–7.

Sackett DL *et al. Evidence-Based Medicine: How to practice and teach EBM.* New York: Churchill Livingstone, 2000.

Applying the evidence

Are your patients similar to those of the study?

How much of the study effect can you expect for your patient or problem?

For Diagnostic tests

Start with your patient's pre-test probability

Pre-test odds = (pre-test probability)/(1 − pre-test probability)

Post-test odds = pre-test odds × LR

Post-test probability = post-test odds/(post-test odds + 1)

For Therapy

Estimate your Patient's Expected Event Rate (PEER)

NNT (for your patient) = 1/(PEER × RRR)

Is the intervention realistic in your setting?

Does the comparison intervention reflect your current practice?

What alternatives are available?

Are the outcomes appropriate to your patient?

Are your patients similar to those of the study?

Of course, your patients weren't in the trial, so you need to apply your clinical expertise to decide whether they are sufficiently similar for the results to be applicable to them. Factors which would affect this decision include:

- The age range included in the trial (many trials exclude the older generations); your group of patients may have a different risk profile, as many drugs have increasing adverse effects in the ageing population which may not be taken into account in the study.
- Many of your patients will have co-morbidity which could affect drug interactions and adverse events as well as benefits.
- Will your patients be able to comply with treatment dosages and duration? For example, compliance might decrease if your patient is taking other medications or if the treatment requires multiple doses daily rather than single ones.
- If NNTs are similar for different treatments, then the NNHs for harmful side effects will become more important; lesser side effects may increase compliance (Bloom, 2001).

The inclusion and exclusion criteria for the study may help as a starting point for your clinical judgment here. It is unlikely, however, that your patient will present an exact match with the study; Sackett *et al* (2000) have recommended framing this question in reverse: How different would your patient have to be for the results of the study to be of no help?

How much of the study effect can you expect for your patient or problem?

To work out how much effect your patient can expect from the intervention, you first need an estimate of their risk of the outcome. This information might be available from a number of external sources, such as cardiovascular risk tables in the British National Formulary, Evidence-based On Call (www.nelh.nhs.uk) or even local audit data. The control group in the study may also provide a good starting point. However, you should use your clinical judgement to arrive at an individual's risk, taking account of his or her individual clinical characteristics.

Diagnosis

In Diagnostic tests, you need to derive an estimate of your patients' pre-test probability, that is the likelihood that they have the disorder prior to doing the test. The prevalance from the study population may act as a guide. Trial data may exist which

> The term **prevalence** is applied to populations, **pre-test probability** is applied to individuals.

generates sensitivities, specificities and LRs for clinical symptoms and signs; see the Rational Clinical Examination series in the *Journal of the American Medical Association*, 1992–2001. This can be combined with the likelihood ratio of the test result to generate a post-test probability.

To calculate a post-test probability, you first need to convert your pre-test probability into pre-test odds (see Altman D, 1991 for more details):

$$\text{Pre-test odds} = (\text{pre-test probability})/(1 - \text{pre-test probability})$$

You can now multiply by the test result's likelihood ratio to yield the post-test odds:

$$\text{Post-test odds} = \text{pre-test odds} \times \text{LR}$$

In turn, these post-test odds can be converted back into a post-test probability:

$$\text{Post-test probability} = \text{post-test odds}/(\text{post-test odds} + 1)$$

However, in the interests of simplicity, we suggest you either use the nomogram on page 24 or the diagnostic calculator at http://cebm.jr2.ox.ac.uk/docs/toolbox.html. The post-test probability from one test can be used as the pre-test probability for the next in a series of independent tests.

Once you have a set of LRs, sensitivities and specificities of the tests you perform, you will quickly see that your post-test probabilities are very much influenced by pre-test probabilities. In the acute setting your clinical judgement will largely determine your patient's pre-test probability. You will see that for low, intermediate and high probabilities, tests vary widely in their usefulness.

Therapy

Two ways of estimating an individual patient's benefit have been suggested by Sackett *et al* (2000).

- **f Method**

This requires that you estimate your patient's risk compared to the control group from the study. Thus, if your patient is twice as susceptible as those in the trial, f = 2; if half as susceptible, f = 0.5. Assuming the treatment produces the same relative risk reduction for patients at different levels of risk, the NNT for your patient is simply the trials reported NNT divided by f.

$$\text{NNT (for your patient)} = \text{NNT}/f$$

Note, however, that if the NNT's confidence intervals are close to the line of no difference, this method becomes less reliable, as it will not detect the point at which those CIs cross the line.

- **Patient Expected Event Rate (PEER) Method**

Alternatively, you could start from an estimate of your patient's risk of an event (expected event rate) without the treatment. This estimate could be based on the study's control group or other prognostic evidence, but you should use your clinical judgement. Multiply this PEER by the RRR for the study: the result is your patient's ARR, which can be inverted to yield the NNT for your patient.

$$\text{NNT (for your patient)} = 1/(\text{PEER} \times \text{RRR})$$

Again, we assume that the same relative benefit would apply to patients at different levels of risk.

Is the intervention realistic in your setting?

You need to consider whether the treatment, test, prognostic factor or causative described in the study would be comparable in your setting, and to what extent any differences would affect your judgement. Amongst the factors you should consider are:

- Did the study take place in a different country, with different demographics?
- Did it take place in a different clinical setting (in-patient, district general, teaching hospital, emergency department, out-patient, general practice)?
- Some interventions, especially diagnostic tests, may be unavailable or slow to come back.
- Will you be able to provide a comparable level of monitoring?
- How you present the treatment options to the patient will be different from the trial; this might significantly affect patient compliance.

Does the comparison intervention reflect your current practice?

If the study compares the benefits of new intervention A with control intervention B, does B match up with what you currently do? If not, you need to think about how your current practice would compare and whether this would affect the extent of any benefit.

Translating an intervention to your practice setting may open up a whole gamut of issues, which we can only touch upon here. However, it is worth asking whether you can adapt your setting. For instance:

- Can your practice nurse develop specialist clinics?
- Can one of your GPs develop a specialist interest?

- Can you introduce protocols which are evidence-based which can be followed by a number of staff, irrespective of seniority?
- Can your guidelines be transferable between different wards or settings?
- How can you maximise your time to make sure that your intervention is realistic in your setting?
- Do your staff need extra training?
- Do your staff need to do a cost-benefit analysis?
- Are you going to audit what you do? Do you need to follow up your patients?

What alternatives are available?

There may be different ways of tackling the same disorder, such as in hypertension, where evidence may be for single or combined drug effects. Again, dosage and delivery are likely to affect compliance, which in turn may make alternatives more practical.

- Have you weighed up the adverse effects of your treatment against those of less helpful treatments? You (or your patient) may feel that a treatment of less benefit which is less harmful may be more appropriate.
- Is doing nothing an option? This relies on your interpretation of the patient's benefits and risk of harm, and what the patient thinks.
- Is there a class effect? Many trials put down the effect to the specific drug and not the generic class.
- Is your patient on so many drugs that it might be worth stopping some or all of them if the adverse effects outweigh the benefits?
- Is your patient aware of lifestyle changes which may be of benefit?

Are the outcomes appropriate to your patient?

What does your patient think? Does your patient understand the implications of the intervention? Some drugs require lifelong adherence to maintain efficacy. The outcomes which are important to you are not necessarily the ones which matter most to your patient, particularly where quality of life is affected. Other important issues to discuss with your patient include:

- Some of the adverse effects may not be mentioned in trials, but may be very relevant to your patient, such as mood disturbances.
- How much reassurance would your patient derive from test results or prognostic estimates?
- The invasiveness of a test or procedure may affect your patient's willingness to participate.
- Implications for further testing and/or treatment.

References

Altman D. *Practical Statistics for Medical Research.* Churchill Livingstone, 1991.
Bloom BS. *Daily regimen and compliance with treatment.* BMJ, 2001;323: 647.
Sackett DL. Straus SE, Richardson WS, Rosenberg W, Haynes RB. *Evidence-Based Medicine: How to practice and teach EBM.* Churchill Livingstone, 2000.

Evidence-based medicine: glossary of terms

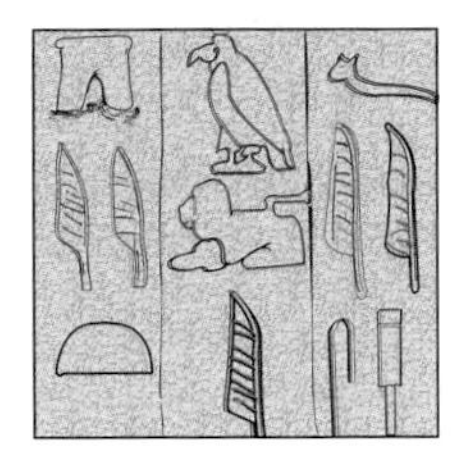

http://cebm.jr2.ox.ac.uk/docs/glossary.html

Absolute risk reduction (ARR): The difference in the event rate between control group (CER) and treated group (EER): ARR = CER – EER. *See p15.*

Adjustment: A summarising procedure for a statistical measure in which the effects of differences in composition of the populations being compared have been minimised by statistical methods.

Association: Statistical dependence between two or more events, characteristics, or other variables. An association may be fortuitous or may be produced by various other circumstances; the presence of an association does not necessarily imply a causal relationship.

Bias: Any tendency to influence the results of a trial (or their interpretation) other than the experimental intervention.

Blinding: A technique used in research to eliminate bias by hiding the intervention from the patient, clinician, and/or other researchers who are interpreting results.

Blind(ed) study (*syn*: masked study): A study in which observer(s) and/or subjects are kept ignorant of the group to which the subjects are assigned, as in an experimental study, or of the population from which the subjects come, as in a non-experimental or observational study. Where both observer and subjects are kept ignorant, the study is termed a **double-blind** study. If the statistical analysis is also done in ignorance of the group to which subjects belong, the study is sometimes described as **triple blind**. The purpose of "blinding" is to eliminate sources of bias.

Blobbogram: *See* Forrest plot.

Case–control study: Involves identifying patients who have the outcome of interest (cases) and control patients without the same outcome, and looking to see if they had the exposure of interest.

Case-series: A report on a series of patients with an outcome of interest. No control group is involved.

CER: Control event rate; *see* event rate.

Clinical practice guideline: A systematically developed statement designed to assist health care professionals and patients make decisions about appropriate health care for specific clinical circumstances.

Cochrane collaboration: A worldwide association of groups who create and maintain systematic reviews of the literature for specific topic areas.

Cohort study: Involves the identification of two groups (cohorts) of patients, one which did receive the exposure of interest, and one which did not, and following these cohorts forward for the outcome of interest.

Co-interventions: Interventions other than the treatment under study that are applied differently to the treatment and control groups. Co-intervention is a serious problem when double blinding is absent or when the use of very effective non-study treatments is permitted.

Co-morbidity: Co-existence of a disease or diseases in a study participant in addition to the index condition that is the subject of study.

Comparison group: Any group to which the intervention group is compared. Usually synonymous with control group.

Confidence interval (CI): The range around a study's result within which we would expect the true value to lie. CIs account for the sampling error between the study population and the wider population the study is supposed to represent. *Around ARR, see p16.*

Confounding variable: A variable which is not the one you are interested in but which may affect the results of trial.

Cost–benefit analysis: Converts effects into the same monetary terms as the costs and compares them.

Cost-effectiveness analysis: converts effects into health terms and describes the costs for some additional health gain (for example, cost per additional MI prevented).

Cost-utility analysis: converts effects into personal preferences (or utilities) and describes how much it costs for some additional quality gain (for example, cost per additional quality-adjusted life-year, or QUALY).

Critically appraised topic (CAT): A short summary of an article from the literature, created to answer a specific clinical question.

Crossover study design: The administration of two or more experimental therapies one after the other in a specified or random order to the same group of patients.

Cross-sectional study: A study that observes a defined population at a single point in time or time interval. Exposure and outcome are determined simultaneously.

Decision analysis: The application of explicit, quantitative methods to analyse decisions under conditions of uncertainty.

Determinant: Any definable factor that effects a change in a health condition or other characteristic.

Dose–response relationship: A relationship in which change in amount, intensity, or duration of exposure is associated with a change – either an increase or decrease – in risk of a specified outcome.

Ecological survey: A study based on aggregated data for some population as it exists at some point or points in time; to investigate the relationship of an exposure to a known or presumed risk factor for a specified outcome.

EER: Experimental event rate; *see* Event rate.
Effectiveness: A measure of the benefit resulting from an intervention for a given health problem under usual conditions of clinical care for a particular group.
Efficacy: A measure of the benefit resulting from an intervention for a given health problem under the ideal conditions of an investigation.
Event rate: The proportion of patients in a group in whom an event is observed. *See p14.*
Evidence-based health care: The application of the principles of evidence-based medicine (see below) to all professions associated with health care, including purchasing and management.
Evidence-based medicine: The conscientious, explicit, and judicious use of current best evidence in making decisions about the care of individual patients. The practice of evidence-based medicine means integrating individual clinical expertise with the best available external clinical evidence from systematic research.
Exclusion criteria: Conditions that preclude entrance of candidates into an investigation even if they meet the inclusion criteria.
f: An estimate of the chance of an event for your patient, expressed as a decimal fraction of the control group's risk (event rate). *See p39.*
Follow up: Observation over a period of time of an individual, group, or initially defined population whose relevant characteristics have been assessed in order to observe changes in health status or health-related variables.
Forrest plot: A diagrammatic representation of the results of individual trials in a meta-analysis.
Funnel plot: A method of graphing the results of trials in a meta-analysis to show if the results have been affected by publication bias.
Gold standard: *see* Reference standard.
Heterogeneity: In systematic reviews, the amount of incompatibility between trials included in the review, whether clinical (ie the studies are clinically different) or statistical (ie the results are different from one another).
Incidence: The number of new cases of illness commencing, or of persons falling ill, during a specified time period in a given population.
Intention-to-treat: Characteristic of a study where patients are analysed in the groups to which they were originally assigned, even though they may have switched treatment arms during the study for clinical reasons.
Interviewer bias: Systematic error due to interviewer's subconscious or conscious gathering of selective data.
Lead-time bias: If prognosis study patients are not all enrolled at similar, well-defined points in the course of their disease, differences in outcome over time may merely reflect differences in duration of illness.
Likelihood ratio: The likelihood that a given test result would be expected in a patient with the target disorder compared to the likelihood that the same result would be expected in a patient without that disorder. *See pp18–20.*

MeSH: Medical Subject Headings: a thesaurus of medical terms used by many databases and libraries to index and classify medical information.
Meta-analysis: A systematic review which uses quantitative methods to summarise the results.
N-of-1 trial: The patient undergoes pairs of treatment periods organised so that one period involves the use of the experimental treatment and one period involves the use of an alternate or placebo therapy. The patients and physician are blinded, if possible, and outcomes are monitored. Treatment periods are replicated until the clinician and patient are convinced that the treatments are definitely different or definitely not different.
Negative predictive value (−PV): The proportion of people with a negative test who are free of disease.
Neyman bias: Bias due to cases being missed because they have not had time to develop or are too mild to be detected at the time of the study.
Number needed to treat (NNT): The number of patients who need to be treated to prevent one bad outcome. It is the inverse of the ARR: NNT = 1/ARR. *See p15.*
Observer bias: Bias in a trial where the measurement of outcomes or disease severity may be subject to bias because observers are not blinded to the patients' treatment.
Odds: A ratio of non-events to events. If the event rate for a disease is 0.1 (10%), its non-event rate is 0.9 and therefore its odds are 9 : 1. Note that this is not the same expression as the inverse of event rate.
Overview: A summary of medical literature in a particular area.
***p* value:** The probability that a particular result would have happened by chance.
PEER: Patient expected event rate: an estimate of the risk of an outcome for your patient.
Placebo: An inactive version of the active treatment that is administered to patients.
Positive predictive value (+PV): The proportion of people with a positive test who have disease.
Post-test probability: The probability that a patient has the disorder of interest after the test result is known.
Pre-test probability: The probability that a patient has the disorder of interest prior to administering a test.
Prevalence: The baseline risk of a disorder in the population of interest.
Prospective study: Study design where one or more groups (**cohorts**) of individuals who have not yet had the outcome event in question are monitored for the number of such events which occur over time.
Publication bias: A bias in a systematic review caused by incompleteness of the search, such as omitting non-English language sources, or unpublished trials (inconclusive trials are less likely to be published than conclusive ones, but are not necessarily less valid).

Randomised controlled clinical trial: A group of patients is randomised into an experimental group and a control group. These groups are followed up for the variables/outcomes of interest.

Recall bias: Systematic error due to the differences in accuracy or completeness of recall to memory of past events or experiences.

Reference standard: A diagnostic test used in trials to confirm presence or absence of the target disorder.

Referral filter bias: The sequence of referrals that may lead patients from primary to tertiary centres raises the proportion of more severe or unusual cases, thus increasing the likelihood of adverse or unfavourable outcomes.

Relative risk (RR) (or risk ratio): The ratio of the risk of an event in the experimental group compared to that of the control group (RR = EER / CER). Not to be confused with relative risk reduction (see below). *See p16.*

Relative risk reduction (RRR): The percentage reduction in events in the treated group event rate (EER) compared to the control group event rate (CER): RRR = (CER−EER) / CER. *See p15.*

Reproducibility (repeatability, reliability): The results of a test or measure are identical or closely similar each time it is conducted.

Retrospective study: Study design in which cases where individuals who had an outcome event in question are collected and analysed after the outcomes have occurred.

Risk: The probability that an event will occur for a particular patient or group of patients. Risk can be expressed as a decimal fraction or percentage (0.25 = 25%).

Risk ratio: *see* Relative risk.

Selection bias: A bias in assignment or selection of patients for a study that arises from study design rather than by chance. This can occur when the study and control groups are chosen so that they differ from each other by one or more factors that may affect the outcome of the study.

Sensitivity: The proportion of people with disease who have a positive test.

Sensitivity analysis: A process of testing how sensitive a result would be to changes in factors such as baseline risk, susceptibility, the patients' best and worst outcomes, etc.

SnNout: When a sign/test has a high sensitivity, a negative result rules out the diagnosis.

Specificity: The proportion of people free of a disease who have a negative test.

Spectrum bias: A bias caused by a study population whose disease profile does not reflect that of the intended population (for example, if they have more severe forms of the disorder).

SpPin: When a sign/test has a high specificity, a positive result rules in the diagnosis.

Stratification: Division into groups. Stratification may also refer to a process to control for differences in confounding variables, by making separate estimates for groups of individuals who have the same values for the confounding variable.

Strength of inference: The likelihood that an observed difference between groups within a study represents a real difference rather than mere chance or the influence of confounding factors, based on both *p* values and confidence intervals. Strength of inference is weakened by various forms of bias and by small sample sizes.

Survival curve: A graph of the number of events occurring over time or the chance of being free of these events over time. The events must be discrete and the time at which they occur must be precisely known. In most clinical situations, the chance of an outcome changes with time. In most survival curves the earlier follow up periods usually include results from more patients than the later periods and are therefore more precise.

Systematic review: An article in which the authors have systematically searched for, appraised, and summarised all of the medical literature for a specific topic.

Validity: The extent to which a variable or intervention measures what it is supposed to measure or accomplishes what it is supposed to accomplish. The **internal validity** of a study refers to the integrity of the experimental design. The **external validity** of a study refers to the appropriateness by which its results can be applied to non-study patients or populations.

Selected evidence-based Healthcare resources on the web

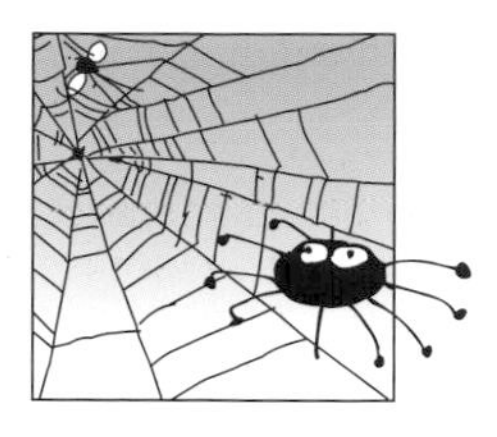

Learning EBM	
Pediatric Critical Care	http://pedsccm.wustl.edu/EBjournal_club.html
University of North Carolina	http://www.hsl.unc.edu/lm/ebm/index.htm
Finding evidence	
CASPfew filters	http://wwwlib.jr2.ox.ac.uk/caspfew/filters/
University of Alberta	http://www.med.ualberta.ca/ebm/ebmtoc.htm
Sources of evidence	
Bandolier	http://www.jr2.ox.ac.uk/bandolier
Best Evidence	http://ebm.bmjjournals.com
Clinical Evidence	http://www.clinicalevidence.org
Cochrane Library	http://www.update-software.com/cochrane
MEDLINE (PubMed)	http://www.ncbi.nlm.nih.gov/entrez/query.fcgi
National Electronic Library for Health (NeLH)	http://www.nelh.nhs.uk
SUMsearch	http://sumsearch.uthscsa.edu/searchform45.htm
TRIP database	http://www.tripdatabase.com
Critical appraisal tools	
CASP	http://www.phru.org/casp/
DISCERN	http://www.discern.org.uk/
Specialties and centres	
Centre for EBM, Toronto	http://www.cebm.utoronto.ca
Centre for Health Evidence	http://www.cche.net
E-B Child Health	http://www.ich.bpmf.ac.uk/ebm/ebm.htm
E-B Dentistry	http://www.ihs.ox.ac.uk/cebd/
E-B Mental Health	http://www.cebmh.com
E-B Nursing	http://www.york.ac.uk/depts/hstd/centres/evidence/cebn.htm
E-B Pharmacotherapy	http://www.aston.ac.uk/pharmacy/cebp/
E-B Social Services	http://www.ex.ac.uk/cebss/
HIRU, McMaster University	http://hiru.mcmaster.ca

Levels of evidence and grades of recommendations

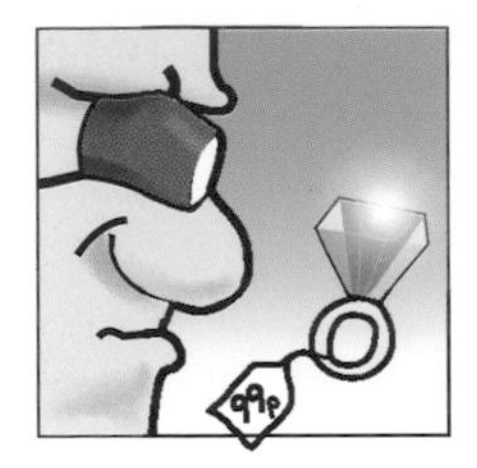

http://cebm.jr2.ox.ac.uk/docs/levels.html

The ancestor of this set of pages was created by Suzanne Fletcher and Dave Sackett 20 years ago when they were working for the Canadian Task Force on the Periodic Health Examination. They generated "levels of evidence" for ranking the validity of evidence about the value of preventive manoeuvres, and then tied them as "grades of recommendations" to the advice given in the report.

The levels have evolved over the ensuing years, have grown increasingly sophisticated, and have even started to appear in a new generation of evidence-based textbooks that announce, in bold marginal icons, the grade of each recommendation that appears in the texts.

However, their orientation remained therapeutic/preventive, and when a group of members of the Centre for Evidence-based Medicine embarked on creating a new-wave house officers' manual (www.eboncall.co.uk), the need for levels and grades for diagnosis, prognosis, and harm became overwhelming and the current version of their efforts appears here. It is the work of Chris Ball, Dave Sackett, Bob Phillips, Brian Haynes, and Sharon Straus, with lots of encouragement and advice from their colleagues.

A final, cautionary note: these levels and grades speak only to the validity of evidence about prevention, diagnosis, prognosis, therapy, and harm. Other strategies, described elsewhere in the Centre's pages, must be applied to the evidence in order to generate clinically useful measures of its potential clinical implications and to incorporate vital patient-values into the ultimate decisions.

Grade	Level of evidence	Therapy/Prevention, Aetiology/Harm	Prognosis	Diagnosis	Economic analysis
A	1a	SR (with "homogeneity") of RCTs	SR (with homogeneity) of inception cohort studies; or a CPG validated on a test set	SR (with homogeneity) of Level 1 diagnostic studies; or a CPG validated on a test set	SR (with homogeneity) of Level 1 economic studies
	1b	Individual RCT (with narrow confidence interval)	Individual inception cohort study with ≥ 80% follow up	Independent blind comparison of patients from an appropriate spectrum of patients, all of whom have undergone both the diagnostic test and the reference standard	Analysis comparing all (critically validated) alternative outcomes against appropriate cost measurement, and including a sensitivity analysis incorporating clinically sensible variations in important variables
	1c	All or none	All or none case-series	Absolute SpPins and SnNouts	Clearly as good or better, but cheaper. Clearly as bad or worse but more expensive. Clearly better or worse at the same cost

Grade	Level of evidence	Therapy/Prevention, Aetiology/Harm	Prognosis	Diagnosis	Economic analysis
	2a	SR (with homogeneity) of cohort studies	SR (with homogeneity) of either retrospective cohort studies or untreated control groups in RCTs	SR (with homogeneity) of Level ≥ 2 diagnostic studies	SR (with homogeneity) of Level ≥2 economic studies
B	2b	Individual cohort study (including low-quality RCT; for example, <80% follow up)	Retrospective cohort study or follow up of untreated control patients in an RCT; or CPG not validated in a test set	Any of: • Independent blind or objective comparison • Study performed in a set of non-consecutive patients, or confined to a narrow spectrum of study individuals (or both) all of whom have undergone both the diagnostic test and the reference standard • A diagnostic CPG not validated in a test set	Analysis comparing a limited number of alternative outcomes against appropriate cost measurement, and including a sensitivity analysis incorporating clinically sensible variations in important variables
	2c	"Outcomes" research	"Outcomes" research		
	3a	SR (with homogeneity) of case–control studies			
	3b	Individual case–control study		Independent blind or objective comparison of an appropriate spectrum but the reference standard was not applied to all study patients	Analysis without accurate cost measurement, but including a sensitivity analysis incorporating clinically sensible variations in important variables

Grade	Level of evidence	Therapy/Prevention, Aetiology/Harm	Prognosis	Diagnosis	Economic analysis
C	4	Case-series (and poor quality cohort and case–control studies)	Case-series (and poor quality cohort and case–control studies)	Any of: • Reference standard was unobjective, unblinded or not independent • Positive and negative tests were verified using separate reference standards • Study was performed in an appropriate spectrum of patients	Analysis with no sensitivity analysis
D	5	Expert opinion without explicit critical appraisal, or based on physiology, bench research or "first principles"	Expert opinion without explicit critical appraisal, or based on physiology, bench research or "first principles"	Expert opinion without explicit critical appraisal, or based on physiology, bench research or "first principles"	Expert opinion without explicit critical appraisal, or based on economic theory

1. These levels were generated in a series of iterations among members of the NHS R&D Centre for Evidence-based Medicine (Chris Ball, Dave Sackett, Bob Phillips, Brian Haynes, and Sharon Straus).
2. Recommendations based on this approach apply to "average" patients and may need to be modified in light of an individual patients unique biology (risk, responsiveness, etc.) and preferences about the care they receive.
3. Users can add a minus sign "–" to denote the level that fails to provide a conclusive answer because of:
   - EITHER a single result with a wide confidence interval (such that, for example, an ARR in an RCT is not statistically significant but whose confidence intervals fail to exclude clinically important benefit or harm)
   - OR a systematic review with troublesome (and statistically significant) heterogeneity. Such evidence is inconclusive, and therefore can only generate Grade D recommendations.
   - By **homogeneity** we mean a systematic review that is free of worrisome variations (heterogeneity) in the directions and degrees of results between individual studies. Not all systematic reviews with statistically significant heterogeneity need be worrisome, and not all worrisome heterogeneity need be statistically significant. As noted above, studies displaying worrisome heterogeneity should be tagged with a "–" at the end of their designated level.

- **CPG** – Clinical practice guideline.
- An **appropriate spectrum** is a cohort of patients who would normally be tested for the target disorder. An inappropriate spectrum compares patients already known to have the target disorder with patients diagnosed with another condition.
- See note #3 above for advice on how to understand, rate and use trials or other studies with wide confidence intervals.
- **All or none**: Met when **all** patients died before the therapy became available, but some now survive on it; or when some patients died before the therapy became available, but **none** now die on it.
- An "Absolute **SpPin**" is a diagnostic finding whose Specificity is so high that a Positive result rules in the diagnosis. An "Absolute **SnNout**" is a diagnostic finding whose Sensitivity is so high that a Negative result rules out the diagnosis.
- **Good, better, bad,** and **worse** refer to the comparisons between treatments in terms of their clinical risks and benefits.
- By poor-quality **cohort** study we mean one that failed to clearly define comparison groups and/or failed to measure exposures and outcomes in the same (preferably blinded), objective way in both exposed and non-exposed individuals and/or failed to identify or appropriately control known confounders and/or failed to carry out a sufficiently long and complete follow up of patients. By poor-quality **case–control** study we mean one that failed to clearly define comparison groups and/or failed to measure exposures and outcomes in the same (preferably blinded), objective way in both cases and controls and/or failed to identify or appropriately control known confounders.
- **By poor-quality prognostic cohort** study we mean one in which sampling was biased in favour of patients who already had the target outcome, or the measurement of outcomes was accomplished in <80% of study patients, or outcomes were determined in an unblinded, non-objective way, or there was no correction for confounding factors.

Study designs

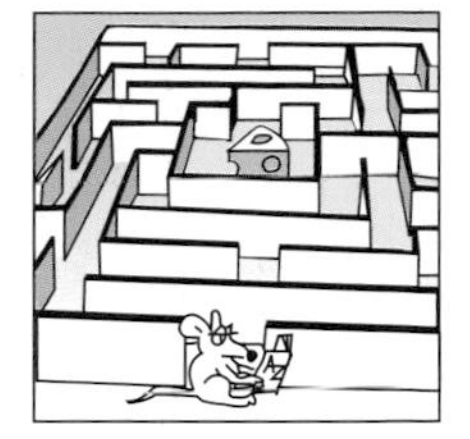

This page gives a brief comparison of the advantages and disadvantages of the different types of study.
http://cebm.jr2.ox.ac.uk/docs/studies.html

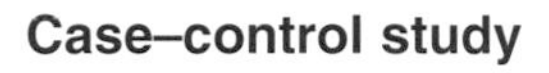

Case–control study

Patients who have developed a disorder are identified and their exposure to suspected causative factors is compared with that of controls who do not have the disorder. This permits estimation of odds ratios (but not of absolute risks).

The advantages of case–control studies are that they are quick, cheap, and are the only way of studying very rare disorders or those with a long time lag between exposure and outcome. Disadvantages include the reliance on records to determine exposure, difficulty in selecting control groups, and in eliminating confounding variables.

Cohort study

Patients with and without the exposure of interest are identified and followed over time to see if they develop the outcome of interest, allowing comparison of risk. Cohort studies are cheaper and simpler than RCTs, can be more rigorous than case–control studies in eligibility and assessment, can establish the timing and sequence of events, and are ethically safe. However, they cannot exclude unknown confounders, blinding is difficult, and identifying a matched control group may also be difficult.

Crossover design

Subjects are randomly assigned to one of two treatment groups and followed to see if they develop the outcome of interest. After a suitable period, they are switched to the other treatment. Since the subjects serve as their own controls, error variance is reduced and a smaller sample size is needed than in RCTs. However, the "washout" period may be lengthy or unknown and crossover designs cannot be used where treatment effects are permanent.

Cross-sectional survey

Measures the prevalence of health factors (outcomes or determinants) at a point in time or over a short period. Cross-sectional studies are relatively cheap and simple to perform, as well as ethically safe. However, they cannot establish causation (only association) and are susceptible to bias (recall bias, confounding, Neyman bias).

Randomised controlled trial (RCT)

Similar subjects are randomly assigned to a treatment group and followed to see if they develop the outcome of interest. RCTs are the most powerful method of eliminating (known and unknown) confounding variables and permit the most powerful statistical analysis (including subsequent meta-analysis). However, they are expensive, sometimes ethically problematic, and may still be subject to selection and observer biases.

Critically appraised topics (CATs)

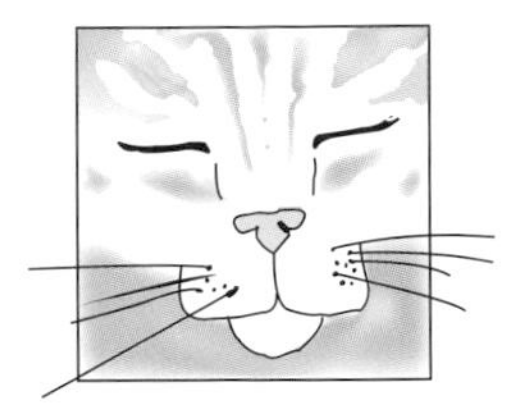

http://cebm.jr2.ox.ac.uk/docs/cats/catabout.html

A CAT is a short summary of the evidence to a focused clinical question. It allows users to store the results of their critical appraisal in such a way that they can easily be shared or stored for later use.

The benefits of CATs

1. They are short and easy to digest.
2. CAT-making fosters the development of EBM skills.
3. They are patient-based and therefore relevant to your practice
4. You can build up a library of CATs which answer common questions.
5. They can be shared.

Potential shortcomings

1. They are a single piece of evidence summarised, not several different pieces of evidence summarised as in a systematic review.
2. They can be wrong.
3. They can quickly become redundant as new evidence becomes available.

You can find some sample CATs at the end of this section.

The key elements of your CAT should be:

1. **Title**. This provides an answer to your question and should be phrased as a declarative statement.
2. **Clinical bottom line**. This is the statement you are making about the paper you are appraising, so you should make sure it is right. If the statement doesn't fit with current practice you should consider whether the evidence you have appraised is of good enough quality to change someone else's or your own practice. If you do think the clinical bottom line is relevant, it may be useful to aid further readers and writers of CATs by making a statement to validate the evidence by looking for further evidence. This can become very relevant when the numbers in trials are low and the confidence intervals are wide. It can also be of benefit to combine papers together in a single CAT, which may support your original findings.
3. **The three-part question**. This records the reason why you went looking for evidence and helps you to re-use the CAT with subsequent questions.
4. **Search terms**. It is important to record how you found the evidence and where. There should be enough detail here to update your search when the CAT's expiry date has been reached.
5. **The study**. In this section, you should include the type of study, number of patients enrolled and their characteristics, exclusion and inclusion criteria, follow up, outcome measures, etc. Be sure to record enough information to allow a reader to decide whether the CAT is of use to them.
6. **The results**. You should include a concise table summarising the evidence (NNT, LRs, ORs, etc). Particularly important here is the selection of which outcome(s) to present: not all the data in the paper will be relevant to your question.
7. **Comments**. These should include any other pertinent issues in the appraisal: the dosages used, side effects, how to implement the procedure, its costs, any other evidence supporting your CAT, etc.
8. **Citation**. So that your conclusions can be checked: if you were planning to change your practice, you would want to check the original data first. You might also like to send your CAT to the trial's author to close the loop between research and practice.
9. **Appraised by and expiry date**. This should include your name and the date on which you appraised the article. The expiry date should be when you think there might be new evidence which supersedes your CAT.

CAT sites on the internet

Centre for Evidence-based Medicine	http://cebm.jr2.ox.ac.uk/docs/catbank.html
Evidence-based On Call	http://www.eboncall.co.uk
University of Michigan Pediatrics	http://www.ped.med.umich.edu/ebm/cat.htm
University of Rochester Medical Center	http://www.urmc.rochester.edu/medicine/res/CATS/index.html
University of Washington	http://depts.washington.edu/pedebm/topic/index.html

Add your own

___

___

___

___

Sample CAT (therapy)

RAMIPRIL REDUCES THE RISK OF DEATH FROM MYOCARDIAL INFARCTION, STROKE AND CARDIOVASCULAR CAUSES IN PATIENTS WITH A HIGH RISK OF A CARDIOVASCULAR EVENT

Clinical bottom line

Treating 26 patients at high risk of a cardiovascular event with Ramipril for at least 5 years will prevent one additional death from myocardial infarction, stroke, and cardiovascular causes.

Citation: HOPE study investigators. Effects of an angiotensin-converting enzyme inhibitor, ramipril, on cardiovascular events in high-risk patients. *N Engl J Med* 2000;**342**:145–53.
Lead author's name and fax: Dr Salim Yusuf, hope@ccc.mcmaster.ca

Three-part clinical question: In a patient at high risk of a cardiovascular event, but without evidence of heart failure, would the angiotensin-converting enzyme inhibitor ramipril reduce their risk of death from cardiovascular causes?
Search terms: Ramipril, angiotensin-converting enzyme inhibitor, heart failure, cardiovascular disease

The study

Non-blinded randomised controlled trial without intention-to-treat.
The study patients: Men and women at least 55 years old, with a history of coronary artery disease, stroke, peripheral vascular disease or diabetes, plus at least one other cardiovascular risk factor (elevated cholesterol levels, low HDL levels, hypertension, documented microalbuminaemia, or cigarette smoking). Patients excluded had heart failure or known low ejection fraction (<0.4), or who were taking an ACE-1, had uncontrolled hypertension or overt nephropathy, or who had had an MI or stroke within 4 weeks of the study beginning.
Control group: (N = 4652; 4652 analysed): Placebo treatment once per day for a mean of five years.
Experimental group: (N = 4645; 4645 analysed): 10 mg ramipril orally once per day for a mean of five years.

The evidence

Outcome	Time to outcome	CER	EER	RRR	ARR	**NNT**
Death from MI, stroke, or CV causes	5 years	0.178	0.14	21%	0.038	**26**
	95% CIs:			13% to 30%	0.023 to 0.053	**19 to 43**
Death from MI	5 years	0.123	0.099	20%	0.024	**41**
	95% CIs:			9% to 30%	0.012 to 0.037	27 to 87
Death from stroke	5 years	0.049	0.034	31%	0.015	**67**
	95% CIs:			14% to 47%	0.007 to 0.023	43 to 145

Comments:
1. Must consider the side effects of ramipril, especially cough, hypotension and dizziness.
2. See the CAT on ramipril for diabetic patients.

Appraised by: Rachael Wright, Corpus Christi College, Oxford, OX1 4JF.; 27 April 2000
Email: rachael.wright@ccc.ox.ac.uk
Kill or Update By: 1 Jan 2001

Sample CAT (diagnosis)

BILIARY TRACT DISEASE: MRCP IS A USEFUL DIAGNOSTIC TOOL

Clinical bottom line

MRCP has a high diagnostic accuracy when compared with direct cholangiography in the detection of biliary tract disease.

Citation: Varghese JC, Farrell MA, Courtney G, Osbourne H, Murray FE, Lee MJ, A prospective comparison of magnetic resonance cholangiopancreatography with endoscopic retrograde cholangiopancreatography in the evaluation of patients with suspected biliary tract disease. *Clin Radiol* 1999;**54:**513–20.
Lead author's name and fax: JC Varghese, Department of Radiology, Beaumont Hospital, Dublin, Ireland.

Three-part clinical question: In a 55-year-old man with jaundice, is magnetic resonance cholangiopancreatography (MRCP) an accurate technique for the diagnosis of biliary trace lesions?
Search terms: In MEDLINE, we searched for magnetic resonance cholangiopancreatography and MRCP and got 225 hits. Limiting the search to clinical trials we got 15 hits, including one up-to-date comprehensive study evaluating the diagnostic accuracy of MRCP as compared with direct cholangiography.

The study

Independent, blind comparison with a reference (gold) standard. There was an appropriate spectrum of patients. The gold standard was applied regardless of the test result.
The study patients: Patients referred with clinical jaundice, abnormal LFTs, biliary colic associated with nausea and vomiting, cholangitis, and gallstone pancreatitis. Patients with contraindications to MRI (cardiac pacemaker, claustrophobia, large size) were excluded, as were patients who had MRCPs of non-diagnostic quality or failed ERCP with no subsequent direct cholangiography.
Target disorder and gold standard: Biliary tract lesions, by direct cholangiography (ERCP, percutaneous transhepatic cholangiography, and intra-operative cholangiography).
Diagnostic test: MRCP using a two-dimensional multi-slice, fast spin echo technique.

The evidence

	Present		Absent			
Test Result	Num.	Prop.	Num	Prop.	LR	95% CI
Positive	28	a	1	b	65.33	0.01 to 458
Negative	2	c	69	d	0.07	0.02 to 0.26
Sensitivity: 93%; CI: 84 to 100				Positive Predictive Value: 97%; CI: 90 to 100		
Specificity: 99%; CI: 96 to 100				Negative Predictive Value: 97%; CI: 93 to 100		
Prevalence: 30%; CI: 21 to 39						

Comments:

1. MRCP is a non-invasive technique in contrast to direct cholangiography. However, a MRCP is a purely diagnostic technique which has no therapeutic capability.
2. The limited availability and cost of MRI currently restricts the use of MRCP to selected centres.

Appraised by: Fenella Pike, Jasmina Cehajic, Caroline Cardy; 3 May 2000
Kill or Update By: May 2001

Index

UMDNJ / Smith-Newark
3 3008 00576 5775